SUPER STRENGTH

THE SECRET TO GAINING STRENGTH - WITHOUT MOVING A MUSCLE

VINCE KOWALSKI

CONTENTS

PREFACE

PREFACE

As a young boy I'd always dreamed of having super strength. I'd play in the backyard of my house and smash my imaginary enemies to oblivion. Yes! Just like the super heroes of my comic books and video games. But alas, it was just a dream, and I knew such things were nonsense.

So, I'd fill the void with conventional weight lifting, and at that time, I would increase my strength quite a bit. In fact, I was squatting 440 pounds at 187 pounds, and deadlifting about 400 pounds. It was hard work and I was constantly eating and having to put on more weight to see the slightest of gains.

Although my strength was much greater than a normal person's, it wasn't what I really wanted, and it was taking up too much of my personal life. Additionally, I'd be constantly tired and in pain. But one night it all changed. I was watching a television series called *Stan Lee's Superhumans*. In the show, it was basically all about Stan Lee (the creator of Marvel comic books) going around the world and documenting people with real-life superpowers.

There were people with super-calculating powers, a real-life samurai that could slice a pellet from a BB gun straight in half! And all sorts of other amazing and wonderful things.

There was one episode that really peaked my interest. It was on man named Dennis Rogers, and he apparently had super strength. He was 5ft 6 and didn't seem like he had a body built for superhuman strength, in fact, he just look liked a regular guy. But to my shock and amazement, I watched this guy first tear a phone book in half like it was nothing, then bend a hammer in half... and he even scrolled up a frying pan! This was incredible, I thought, this guy literally had super strength. Although the episode concluded, he was genetically a freak... he had to be. That was my take on it, for sure. But, after I did some researching on Dennis a little more, I realized this was not the case, and that he had actually been training in a special method, a lost and forgotten training. I also came to learn that there had been so many more before him with similar (if not greater) feats of strength achieved.

So, this is where it all started for me, and I guess that's what this book is all about. Right now, I'm going to share with you my research, the history, and the magnificence of the people behind the reality of how to literally bend steel with your bare hands... and so much more! Thanks so much for joining me here.

1

THE SECRET KEY TO SUPER STRENGTH

THE MAJOR KEY HERE IS *ISOMETRICS*. IF THERE WERE ANY REAL secrets in the world of super strength, this is definitely the be-all and end-all. When done properly, using isometrics gets you past any plateau which can be the difference between ongoing success or failure. A highly underestimated tool, it's no wonder it is one of the most negated forms of strength training. But... those that know this powerful secret, hold the wisdom to unlock true, superhuman potential, or powers.

Remaining focused is the most important aspect of any exercise system. And whether it's muscle control, lifting weights, rep training, or even going for extended periods of time in one exercise form, the difference remains the same. Yes, isometrics really takes on an exceptionally new level of focus, and a much-needed, perfected concentration level that is accurate and on point. It doesn't matter if you hold a position for 12 seconds or 12 hours, the focus is still required. It takes monumental focus and concentration, and not just within the physical body, but also internally as a focal point of belief. The real secret with isometrics is not how long you can hold any posture, position or contraction... the real power is in how much internal power you can attain and hold for the period of integration. This *IS* the secret.

One of the world's (quite possibly the greatest) renowned wrestlers, The Great Gama, was a testament to the sport as an incredible athlete. In fact, Gama was well-known for his unbelievably-brutal workout training, ranging from swimming right through to wrestling. He even did some exercises for hours on end. Additionally, the massive amount of repetitions he achieved for both push-ups and squats were phenomenal. On a global scale, he was famous for never losing a match in his entire career, which was 5000 matches in total. An unbelievable human being.

Gama was fierce with both his renowned takedown and throwing techniques, and he could toss his opponents without any real effort, or so it seemed. Part of his training entailed tying a belt or a strap around a tree. He would then try with every ounce of his strength and internal focus to take down that tree. Gama also incorporated other forms of isometrics too, and his opponents were not really excited about facing him in the wrestling ring, for understandable reasons. He was fierce and all-powerful. We will touch on him some more, soon, a little later in the title.

It's important to understand that the major practice of isometrics is best done by working them into your own training regimen, or just doing them as they were intended. This is because, great practice methods that (historically) work, have already been researched and trialed well, so we know that they can create the success we seek. If you can stay open-minded, you'll find yourself in a wonderful new world of strength training. One that's more successful, healthier, and much more efficient to your body's needs, as opposed to the weight machines, cardio machines, and the vast array of dumbbells you see being utilized these days. So yes, we can find a unique methodology of real strength training and great, purposeful ability from some of the greats. The ones who did it for real, historically. We'll take a look at them soon, so stay tuned for that.

Prior to weight lifting equipment and the ushering in of up-to-date gyms, individuals who sought to increase size and strength used to push against stationary objects. A straightforward way to see this is by locking your hands together and pushing back against yourself with as much force as possible.

To simplify the fact, muscles only contract in specific ways. One of the most obvious ways is when contracting and shortening the muscle lengths when doing bicep curls. The technical term for this is concentric contraction, and this is where muscles tense while they contract (shorten in length).

Muscles are also able to tense while they lower loads (or resist against them). This would occur when dropping the arm back to the starting position in a bicep curl. This contraction type is termed eccentric, and this arises as the muscle becomes tense as it lengthens.

Another muscle contraction is known as an isometric contraction which occurs when the muscles tense without any change in their length. Prime examples are when body-building posing or when pushing against objects which are immovable, such as walls.

Isometric training possesses the main benefits where the body can activate almost all of the available motor units to some degree; this is typically, extremely hard to accomplish.

Way back during the 1950s, scientists Hettinger and Muller established a single daily effort of around two-thirds of a person's possible maximum. When exerted for a period of only six seconds at a time, and performed over a ten week period, strength increased by around 5% each week.

Clark and associates established that static strength carried on increasing, even after a five-week regimen of isometric exercises had concluded.

Additional benefits of isometric training are purely the total time spent performing any given exercise. When considering exercises like bench presses, it might take one or two seconds to perform the action for each joint angle. Each muscle only needs training for reduced periods of time.

On the contrary, exercises which mimic bench presses, such as a press against pins at the locking position of a lift, well, these might need to be performed for more than a few seconds. What this means is, if you find you have problems at specific joint angles during your lift, you can use targeted isometrics which helps to alleviate your problems, right then and there.

Typically, as soon as we raise weights, our muscles absorb type-2 fiber. It is once we start approaching our maximum effort of 100% that the body forces itself to engage its fast-twitch muscle fibers. If this were not to happen, these would then become neglected. When training in this nature, we see results in increased strength as micro-tears are created in the most powerful cells in the muscles, and which increase as they heal. Amazing!

To fully use 100% effort, we have only two techniques in which we can use. Either we can lift 100% of our one rep maximum capacity, or we can lift around 85% of maximum capacity, but with increased speed and explosiveness. This varies to our regular exercises, with the lifting of heavy weights and employing bursts of explosive speed. This requires the body to generate additional force. It is this occur-rence that helps our muscle strength increase.

Holding weights in position until we feel a complete fatigue is an alternative way of movement. And this utilizes the fast-twitch muscle fibers of the body, as it does when you push or pull against an object which you are unable to move. When merely pushing or pulling against an object which you are unable to move, ultimately your body starts adapting to be in the condition to move this object over time. Additionally, this also goes a long way to create stronger "neural drives" between the brain and muscles. And as it happens, when you command your body to use all of its muscle, you then also increase the ability to engage muscle fiber at will. Feedback is also forthright as you start feeling that your muscles are working. As fast-twitch muscle fibers are the most significant type, these are the best to increase hypertrophy and show a visible increase in muscle size.

2

HOW STRONG CAN WE
REALLY GET?

At the beginning of the 20th century, the world started to see the introduction of a previously unseen kind of public hero: professional strongmen. These strongmen arose from physical culture movements which were built during the 1800s as a response to what we now know as the Industrial Revolution.

With the explosion of office working, there was an increasing concern in what way this new deskbound lifestyle was affecting overall health — and "manliness," for the men of the nation.

Strongmen became symbols of preserved virility, and living proof the male citizens still possessed grit, power, and the strength of their ancestors, with the potential for performing macho, or masculine activities. If men were no longer able to tame the wild frontier, and face the challenges of nature, they, in turn, could become masters of themselves, and then pit their resoluteness against the weights and feats of the strength of a gymnasium.

And so, strongmen arrived from all corners of the world, and diverse cultural backgrounds, too. Some materialized from the ranks of professional and amateur athletes. They were previously boxers, wrestlers, or participants in the Olympics (and the lesser-known Highland games).

Some previously served as physical training instructors in the military forces, while others had merely been in laborious jobs like those of blacksmiths or factory laborer positions. Here, they saw the chance to make a decent living by using their brawn in a less tedious and grueling way.

Strongmen found no shortage of where to ply their trade. Even displaying feats of strength and prowess in floor show acts, which were performed in music halls and the many dime-store museums. The lifting of these heavy weights as an end, was in fact, an unusual-enough concept, and so it grabbed the attention of, and captivated the public audiences. They were willing to pay to watch powerfully-built men hoist dumbbells, barbells, and other peculiarly-formed objects.

Strongmen broadened their acts while incorporating stunts. The barehanded breaking of chains, tearing decks of cards in half, and bending iron bars and horseshoes. This was the leadup to pulling large items by only their teeth, and also engrossing the crowds with mock gladiatorial tournaments.

Many deceptions were performed in these shows. With entertainers using trickery and deception to pull off their perceptible deeds of strength. Nonetheless, there were genuine strength participants on the show circuits, who did insist that it was to be manpower alone when performing their lifts and stunts.

These strongmen turned out to be, not only the promoters of engaging sideshows, but they also aided to evolve an awareness of physical cultures and overall fitness to a broader public audience. Naturally, regular men wanted to know how they too could build similar physiques, especially after seeing these strongmen perform.

A number of these strongmen went on to create numerous books and mail-order courses. These courses laid out the suggested strength-building programs. They remained immensely available in the first half of the 20th century. Such was the impact; they helped to launch a fitness (awareness) culture which still remains as a part of our history, even today.

Some of the acts that strongmen performed involved many classic lifts and exercises. A number of these are still recognized today (although much of what is considered good form has been improved over time), like the squat, jerk and clean, and more. Some other exercises were truly unique and have now mostly-been forgotten since the zenith of these old-time strongmen.

If the effects of isometric training still don't have you convinced, then ponder over the thought for a moment, it is the foundation of some of the world's strongest people ever born. They realized their abilities and capabilities by utilizing isometrics.

How strong can we really become? Well, when talking about some of the legendary strongmen feats, you can quickly get the idea of how amazing our bodies are and what they really can achieve.

3

STRONGMAN HALL OF FAME

ALEXANDER ZASS – THE IRON SAMSON

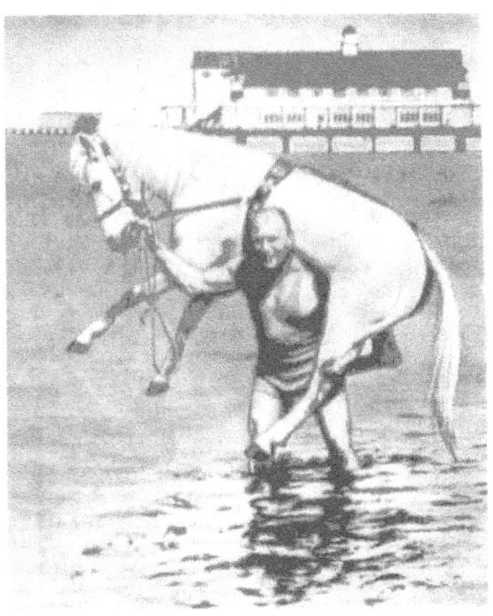

1888 - 1962

Alexander Zass was born in Vilna, Poland. However, he spent his younger years living in Russia. Like countless other strongmen of his period, Zass was driven to increase his strength after attending a circus and seeing the exploits performed by the circus strongman there.

Zass began with the bending of green branches, climbing trees and running with his home-made dumbbells and barbells. It was later that he trained beneath some of the most-famous, professional, Russian strongmen.

Zass developed incredible strength which allowed him to transport a horse on his shoulders. His most momentous talents were the bending of steel bars and the breaking of chains, which became the centerpiece of his exhibitions.

Interesting Fact: In 1914, while he served in the Russian army at some stage in the First World War, Zass became wounded and was taken prisoner by Austrian forces. As a prisoner of war, he persistently developed his strength by using isometrics. He did this by pulling on the bars and chains. Zass ultimately escaped from his prison and never returned to his homeland.

Out of all the strongmen, he is without a doubt, my favorite. There are a few old black and white videos of him performing some of his crazy feats. Click here if you want to have a look.

"I aimed first, to develop the underlying connective tissues rather than the superficial muscles. I developed tendon strength. The tendons are the cord-like media between the bones and the muscles. A large bicep is no more criterion of strength than a swollen abdomen is of digestion. It is the pulling tendon of the biceps that counts. Moreover, so on throughout the whole body, this method was employed. Some men with thin legs are stronger than some with thick legs. Why? Because strength lies in the tendons; they are the powerful fibrous attachments of the muscles to the bones. They are, in short, the master key to the strength which overcomes great resistance. Without tendons, one

would possess no control over the body. There would be no rigidity, no steadiness of physical movement. They, and their development, are the secret of my strength. I am tendon-strong. Muscles alone won't hold horses back. Tendons will; and do. But they must be cultivated. Oh, yes. They must be developed. There is a way of increasing their strength, and that way, I claim in all modesty, I have perfected. Real, sound, and efficient is my method." - Alexander Zass

Siegmund Breitbart

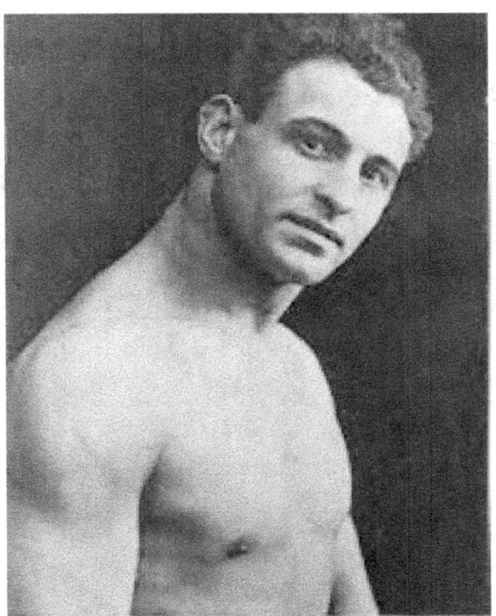

1883 - 1925

Breitbart made his performances expansively around Europe and America while he toured with the Circus Busch. He did this by molding a strength act which was themed to fit in with his former career as a blacksmith. He went on to bend iron bars around his arms. These, he did in floral patterns before he bit through iron chains, or ripped them apart, and even tore horseshoes in half.

As a complete showman, Breitbart's feats also came to include the holding back of two whipped horses or being able to pull a wagon-load of people by using only his teeth. He was also seen supporting huge weights, such as vehicles that were laden with up to ten passengers.

Stones were broken by sledge hammers on his chest all while he was lying on his back, and he also picked up a baby elephant. While he held the elephant, he climbed up a ladder and then held a locomotive wheel using a rope (using his teeth). If this was not enough, three men sat suspended from the locomotive wheel.

Breitbart took the most famous feats that other strongmen performed in his era and made it a significant part of his act, too. For the duration of The Tomb of Hercules, a bridge was constructed over his chest. Massive beasts such as bulls or elephants were paraded across the boards.

Breitbart, however, took it a stage further. He took to supporting a motordrome on his chest. At this point, two men followed each other on the inside while riding motorcycles.

I liked his method of isometric training much more than any other. It involved the increasing of the weight on any given exercise, by way of increments. Doing this day by day is done so as not to lose any energy. Furthermore, by doing so, his body continually adapted to the weight increases without tiring himself out!

Checkout this video on his feats

Dennis Rogers

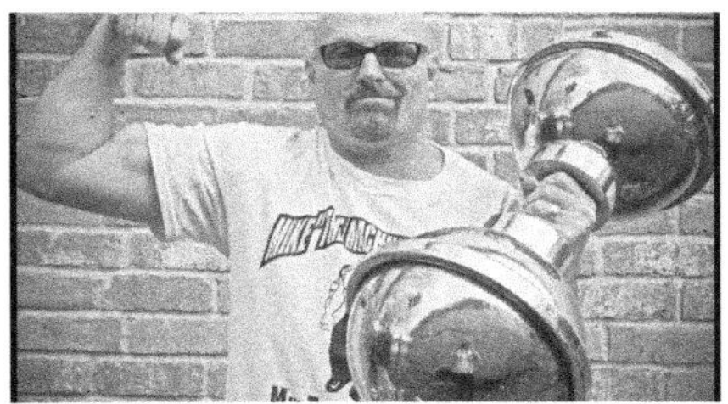

1958 - present

Any modern-day Hercules who can rip telephone books into two and who bends steel wrenches and hammers with his hands is simply amazing. A mountain of a man. Standing at 5 feet 6 inches and only weighing 168 pounds, Dennis Rogers appears like an average 60-year-old. He is still considered to be the pound-for-pound, world's strongest man.

Dennis Rogers weighed 80 pounds when he was entering high school. He appeared too frail, so he was admitted into a *special education* gym class. At this point, he believed he'd never be large enough to do anything sports-related during his entire life.

Nevertheless, in the early 70s, something transformed in Dennis' insight about who he was, and the things he was capable of doing. Dennis remembers his brothers, and he watched a television program about a man who tore a deck of cards in two. They then drove to the closest store to purchase a pack of cards, and so they, themselves, could try the trick.

Dennis sat in the driver's seat as his brother handed him the pack, he held it and tore it apart on the first attempt. That was the first time he realized he was capable of much more than what he previously thought. Since that time, Dennis Rogers (among other things) became World Arm-Wrestling Champion and a Grandmaster Strongman, who was capable of bending steel hammers and wrenches, and could even stop an aircraft from taking off... with his bare hands!

Heres a cool video of him showing of his strength

Bruce Lee

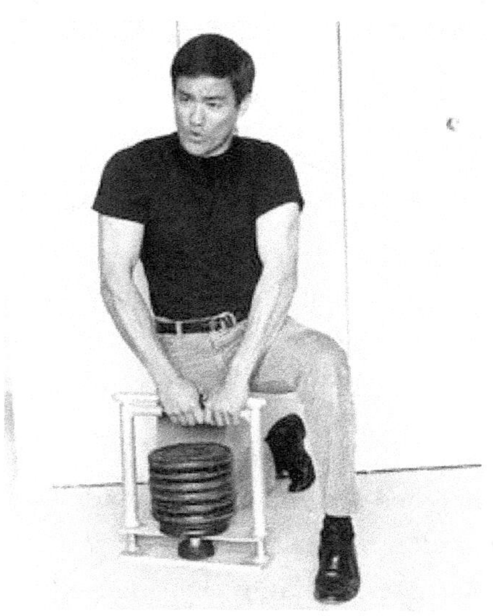

1940 - 1973

Bruce Lee? That's right; even the great Bruce Lee knew the possibilities and the secrets of isometric training. As an example, he used isometric training and was capable of nailing a steel chain to the floor. To this, he attached a bar, and then he would try to 'curl' the bar.

Supplementary exercises he used frequently, involved the holding of himself in a gymnastic 'V-sit' position. He would then hang from a bar where he would raise his legs and hold.

Lee understood and believed in the importance of the "neural drive" we mentioned earlier. He trained this by using static contractions – the tensing of his muscles.

Lee always made sure he tensed his entire body throughout his exercises. This, he said, was to plug energy leaks and was how he managed to perform the famous "one finger push up." He used the contractions at each end of the muscle. This increased mind-muscle connections while increasing his *time under tension.*

Lee's training involved so much isometric training. He used the methodology to build and improve his physique, as well as his incredible strength and power. Furthermore, as a reminder of how strong Bruce Lee was – he was the guy who was able to hold an 88-pound (40 kg) barbell at arm's length. He could then hold this position for a number of seconds, seemingly effortlessly. What an absolute legend.

The Great Gama

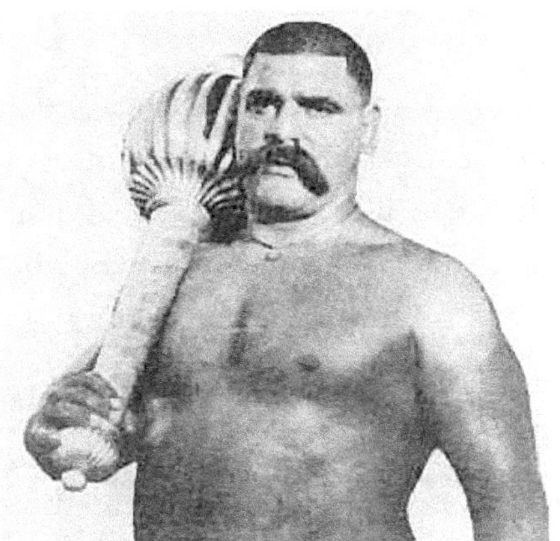

1878 - 1960

Gama apparently attributed a significant portion of his incredible power to the use of isometric training, too. One of his more-renowned workouts involved the tying of a rope around a tree while trying to pull the tree over. This training helped him to develop his incredible strength, and it is also one of the coolest training techniques you are likely to ever hear of... pretty cool!

The Great Gama or Ghulam Muhammad, was a wrestler and a strongman who was born in 1878 in the then, "British India." He was better known for his long and very successful wrestling career. He remained reigning for over 50 years. His training methods, and the feats of strength he performed also started to play a role in his popularity.

Ghulam's father trained him, he was also a successful wrestler, and at a very young age, the general public noticed Ghulam too. He appeared at a strongman competition at the tender age of 10. The competition had more than 400 participants, which featured a large number of harsh exercises, such as Indian squats. Ghulam Muhammad fortified his place among the final fifteen wrestlers. Subsequently, as he showed such incredible devotion and commitment for his age, The Great Gama was announced the winner of the competition.

Within nine years, The Great Gama broadcasted a challenge against the Indian wrestling champion (who at the time, was Raheem Baksh). He was much taller than him at 6'9" while Gama himself stood at 5'7" being significantly smaller. Imagine the height and reach advantage Raheem had against Ghulam in this match!

The Great Gama succeeded and won the match, which marked a turning point in his career. There were many other, well-known wrestlers like Stanislaus Zbysko, Dr. Benjamir Roller, Maurice Deriaz, and John Lemm, who all fell to the same fate of loss against Ghulam.

The Great Gama traveled to Baroda at the age of 22. He went to compete in wrestling. Unhappily, he couldn't find a match; he then decided to try something else. He raised 1200 kg (2645 pounds) onto his chest and then dropped it down after he carried it for a period. It was 2.5 feet in height, and it is still kept at Baroda Museum for display.

Gama's diet included (daily) drinking 2 gallons of milk mixed with 1.5 pounds of paste made from crushed almonds and fruit juice. He trained on a daily basis, and he performed 3000 Hindu pushups coupled with 5000 Hindu squats. The squats he performed while he wore 200 pounds of apparatus, and then he would ask that someone rub him down with dry mustard after each workout session.

One other interesting fact about this great man, is the significant influence he had on many. Bruce Lee being one of them. Once he read about Gama's extraordinary strength, Bruce decided to integrate Gama's training approaches into his exercise routine. This might have helped him to achieve his legendary status. The Great Gama, unfortunately, died in 1960 after losing the fight with a long history of heart-related conditions.

Eugen Sandow

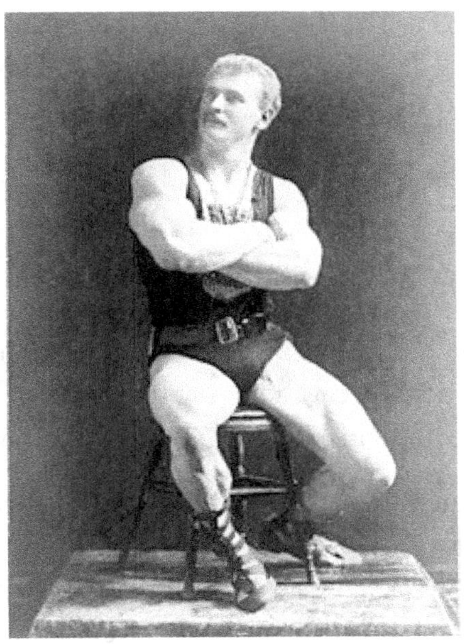

1867 - 1925

He has often been called *The Father of Modern Bodybuilding*. Eugen Sandow was a traveling, performing strongman. He showed the country incredible feats of strength which included the bearing of the weight of horses and soldiers on his chest. He snapped chains, bent iron bars, lifted pianos, and even bench pressed a cow. Wow!

He was also well-known for his acrobatic athleticism; he was able to perform a back somersault while holding a 50 lb. dumbbell in both hands. One feat of strength was his bench press capability of 300 pounds.

The majority of Sandow's training involved heavy dumbbell and heavy barbell weightlifting:

"My faith has always been pinned to dumbbells. I do all my training using them and supplement this training with weightlifting (with barbells)." – Eugen Sandow

Due to their reduced size, it is conceivable to have a vast dissimilarity in the weight of dumbbells, rather than the longer-handled bar known as the barbell (back then, barbells were fixed in weight and were not adjustable).

Any physical individual can acquire numerous pairs of dumbbells and be in a position to gradually practice more while training. Weight lifting using barbells can add a variety of interest and benefit to any training program. The most substantial and dominant muscles of the legs and back are brought into action with the heavy barbell. This can be done through competitive or exhibition lifting as a sport.

All the exercises should be accomplished gradually for the muscles to accustom themselves to the work they need to perform. If the demand is not increasingly made more substantial, the anticipated increase in size, strength, and shape will never be accomplished.

Sandow was well-known for lifting lighter dumbbells during his training, while still achieving excellent results. The reason for this being, he implemented what we know today as the *mind-muscle connection.*

When he lifted lighter dumbbells. Sandow did not only go through the gestures; he focused on employing as many motor units as was conceivable with every muscle contraction.

"You might go through a list of exercises using dumbbells a hundred times a day. Unless your mind is fixed on those muscles where the work is to be applied, any such exercise would bear little, if any, benefit.

If you concentrate your mind on the muscles you are using, then you will immediately see development begins." - Eugen Sandow

Sandow also employed some form of scheduling into his training, and always varied the intensity:

"Variation in your training program will always bring best the results. Don't train every day. It is better to skip a day now and then, so the muscles have time to rest thoroughly. This gives nature the opportunity to reconstruct the muscles while building their strength and endurance.

You should never train with the identical weight. Vary the days, and for some, use more modest weights which help tone muscles. On the other training days, really push yourself. Here, you can give your muscles plenty of work to do. Nature can then take care of building strength, more muscle, and overall better health." – Eugen Sandow

The above examples are just a handful of the amazing, magnificent people and their feats who benefited from using isometrics. And, through their scope and adaptation of technique, their significance as strongmen does an excellent job to show how isometrics can improve strength and also how you can look like a demi-god in the process. And all from practicing techniques using isometrics as a must-do method of training!

For Your Program

It is my belief that these energetic days should not be performed by an ordinary man more than once or twice a week. I go through my program up to four times a day. This depends on my schedule. However, after years of progressive training and living healthily, this has led to my ability in being able to withstand such a rigorous program while continuing to gain strength and enhancement. All the while, still preserving perfect health. This is detrimental.

4

WHY?

WHY ISN'T THIS COMMON KNOWLEDGE?

The fact that you can perform useful isometrics with very little equipment and in a relatively short period of time, should be vocalized more-publicly. You would think more individuals would be aware of it, and that they would become more popular in the training world by doing so.

So why are isometrics not mainstream?

For starters, there is the commercial aspect. Anything that can lose companies' money will always get pushed to the back of 'the line.' Isometrics are no different, because there is really no valuable equipment needed, so there is little for these companies to benefit from.

Secondly, there is the selective use of the science involved in isometric research. No point backing something that won't make loads of cash. Sad but true.

5

7 REASONS YOU NEED RADICAL HAND STRENGTH

I MADE A FUNDAMENTAL OBSERVATION OVER THE YEARS regarding the bulk of men who work out. They disregard the importance of training with the hands. Keeping this in mind, I thought I'd go through and swiftly list a few reasons you should build your own incredible hand strength.

1 – Your hands lead the body. From the messages the nervous system sends your body, it actually thinks your hands are enormous. They contain twice the number of nerve endings compared to other parts of the body. When you exercise and train your hands to be strong, you are, in fact, helping to condition your nerves. This nerve force is a fundamental component of health and strength, and it was definitely a massive factor for the old-time strongmen of yesteryear.

2 – The hands help to make more of your physical power useable. You will have the ability to lift heavier weight using your back, legs, and shoulders too. This applies to the more significant muscle groups of the body. Unfortunately, what stops many people in the real

world, is the lack of strength in their hands. If you can generate 500 lbs. of force with your legs and back, but your hands can only accommodate 300 lbs., then you inefficiently limit yourself in the real world, which is unfortunate, but true.

3 – Hand's help to stimulate the entire body. Again, we traverse back to the nerves. Most movements we perform in the old-time strongman tradition show us that hand training helps to stimulate the body. If you aspire to increase health, more muscle, more strength, then it's necessary. It's time to kick your body into gear from a nerve and hormonal point of view. The hands have to be trained hard with immense exercises that give the whole body a workout.

4 – Many hand exercises aid in building serious muscle. Take a look at two of the top students of the old-time arts - Mike "The Machine" and Bruce and Pat "The Human Vise" Povilaitis – Both possess enormous muscular development. Now, do they do other forms of training? They do, absolutely, yes. However, they also perform lots of bending, and this is BIG bending! When this is implemented well, this bending works several muscles inside, and these small muscles you are unable to see. If you wish to build some serious muscle and make sure it's a muscle that's fully functional, make sure to work your hands with strongman training.

5 – Your hand strength is able to save lives! It is quite sad to know that there are a lot of people who cannot pull themselves over a wall. This could be out of the way of a flood, an emergency situation that could require a quick exit from an area, or any other life-threatening situation. A large part of the reason is due to great hand strength, and if hands are too weak, then they will (subsequently) let an individual down. Most modern society activities do not need exceptional hand strength. Nevertheless, that should not stop you possessing what you ought to have. Tremendous hand strength, and the natural ability to use those hands in ways that are practical is paramount. And in ways that can literally save people's lives.

6 – For self-defense. A vast number of people think the modern world is safer than it actually is. Let's be truthful – there are places around the world, even in America, that are nowhere close to being safe. The stronger you can make your hands, the better chance you have to defend yourself and that of a partner or family member.

You need strong hands! By training with the strongman feats in the same way, this is one of the best ways for building hand strength. It is a fact, and it's not only a great way of increasing hand strength, but you will also find you can have a lot of fun in the process. At the end of it, you will have the great sense of accomplishment, too.

6

GETTING STARTED WITH ISOMETRICS

THERE ARE THREE COMMONLY KNOWN ISOMETRIC METHODS.

1. Static Tension
2. Muscle against Muscle
3. Forcing Yourself Against Immovable Objects

Max Sick Utilized Static Tension for Increased Greater Control & Development

Max Sick, born on the 28th of June, in 1882, in Württemberg, Germany. He was very ill from a very young age with severe lung difficulties, dropsy, and rickets. At 5 years of age, he couldn't even stand on his own two feet. In fact, the doctors informed his family that each year he got older, the chances of Max surviving would become slimmer and slimmer.

Aged 10, Max made his own weights. He then developed his own exercise routine. Conversely, his parents were intensely in disagreement to him weight lifting, and actually threw them into the trash.

Yet, Max as determined as ever to develop his body, formed a sequence of muscle control workouts. By 14 years of age, he had made such an improvement in his development, he was asked if he wished to join a local athletics club.

The isometrics methods Max created were a variety of *Static Tension Isometrics*. When performing these isometrics, you flex your muscles with no joint movement. The secret is contracting each muscle group as hard as is achievable.

Max Sick's Physical Feats:

- Max could make his many groups of muscles spasm in time to music.
- Max could press a man 40 pounds heavier than he was, above his head, for up to 16 reps.

Charles Atlas Put "Muscle Against Muscle" For Increased Strength

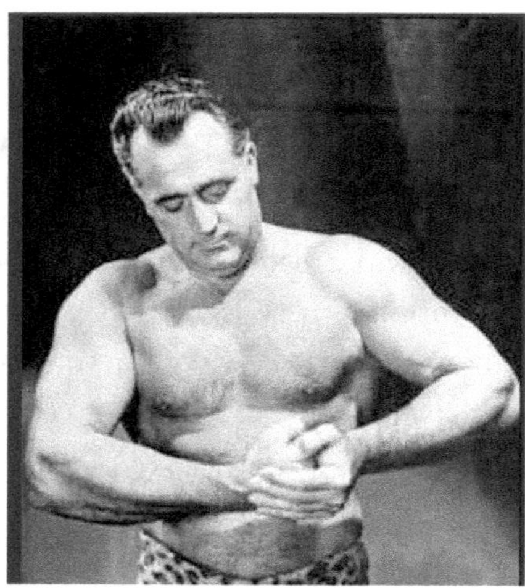

Charles Atlas went from a 'scrawny weakling' to become one of the most popular musclemen in modern history. He was born "Angelo Siciliano," but later changed his name to Charles Atlas. This came from his friend who said that the Atlas statue (that sat on the Coney Island Hotel) looked like him.

Charles developed his system of exercises called "Dynamic Tension." Here, you put "muscle against muscle" and use your own muscular force which generates fatigue. These isometrics are looked at as "sister exercises," along with Dynamic Tension and are called, "Yielding Isometrics."

Fundamentally, you place your hands and feet in specific locations and push against each other as hard as you are able to.

Charles Atlas' Physical Feats:

- He could tear a telephone book and deck of cards into two.
- He was able to bend (double) a 6-inch spike.

- He was able to smash a 3 and a 1/2-inch nail through sturdy pine planks (up to 2 inches).
- He could easily bend a steel bar that was 6 feet in length and 1/2 an inch in thickness.
- He could drag an automobile with only his neck.
- One end of a vehicle could be clearly lifted off the ground.
- Charles could raise a pony into the air.

Alexander Zass Established Incredible Power by Exerting Himself against Immobile Objects

Alexander Zass was born in Vilnius. He was a circus actor who went on to be a professional wrestler and then a successful strongman. He had remarkable strength and was able to break chains, bend thick bars, and to carry a small horse on his shoulders.

He was well known for the ability to catch a 90 kg cannon ball which was fired from a cannon. Zass generated his own style of isometric exercises and practiced them even when he was a POW after being captured by Austrian forces during WWI.

He escaped on three occasions and left the country after his third attempt. While in prison, he practiced his style of isometrics called, "Overcoming Isometrics." This method pulls and pushes against fixed objects. The object is to create the most considerable amount of force as is possible. Because the object that you are pulling or pushing against is immobile, you are able to force your body's muscles to full capacity.

Alexander Zass' Physical Feats:

- The ability to break shackles and bend thick iron bars (this is how he managed to escape from prison).
- He was able to carry a full piano strapped to his back with people sat on top.
- He was able to snap smaller trees in half.

7

STRONGMAN EXERCISES

So lets get started. Theses are some exercises i've pulled from some of my favourite strongman books. As you can see they're easy to do, require little to no equipment and take very little amount of your time.

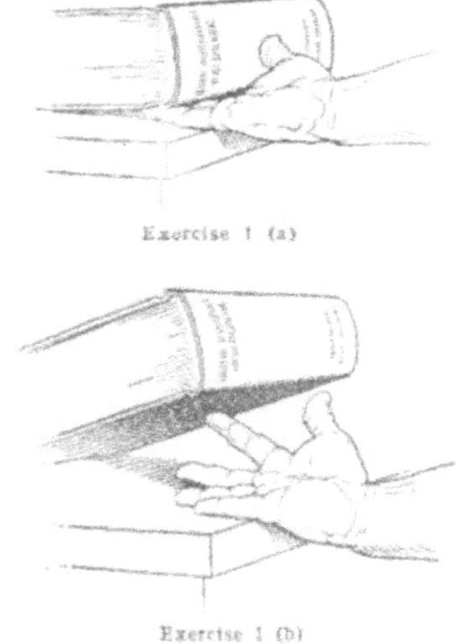

Exercise 1 (a)

Exercise 1 (b)

Finger Extensions: Exercise 1 (a)

1. You'll be surprised to find how weak your fingers are, at first. It's important to use a book of a fairly good weight.
2. You will notice that the book is placed on the fingers (only) and it is not touching the hand at all. Additionally, note that the hand is not resting on the table. These two points are important. Allowing the back or the palm of the hand to rest will defeat the purpose of the exercise, here.

Exercise 1 (b)

1. When you have raised the book to your limit, you will need to lower it back to the first position.
2. Now, position and focus doing the same with the next finger, until every finger on both of your hands has been

done. An exercise for the thumb comes a little later on. So, leave the thumb out for this one.

3. It's important to practice raising the book with each finger several times, before moving to the next digit.

4. After you have completed the exercises individually, now try raising the book with your digits, one after the other, as quickly as possible. This will help form speed and strength.

Reverse Finger Extensions: Exercise 2

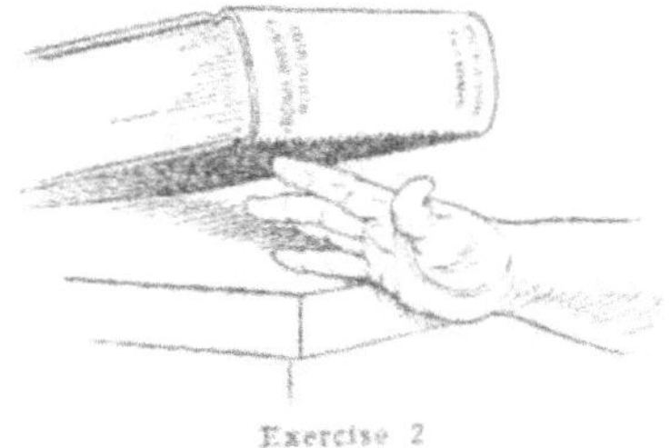

Exercise 2

1. Go through the same process as explained for the first exercise, utilizing the fingers individually, and then quickly, afterward.

2. The only major change in action in this movement is, that you are requiring more care than in the first exercise. This is reversed, too.

3. As your fingers move individually to the small finger, a natural inclination will be felt to move the thumb. Helping to strengthen it as you go.

8

BROOM EXTENSION TECHNIQUE

EXERCISE 4

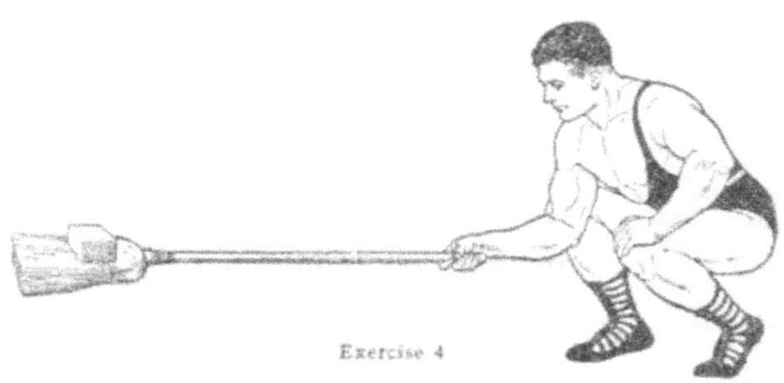

1. At first, you'll practice with a broom on its own.
2. When holding the end of the broom, simply move the hand down the handle and shorten the leverage. Do this if you find it difficult to hold the end, at first. And as you grow in strength, you can move the hand grip further, toward the end of the handle. Over time, it will get easier.
3. When this is accomplished, over a period of time, you may add more weight on, by placing an object on the straw end of the broom, as is shown in the picture.

4. It is important that the broom is in a straight line with the forearm, and neither the elbow or the arm can rest (against or) upon the knee. The entire arm must be free and act independently of any other aid or support.

BARREL DIGITING

Barrel Digiting

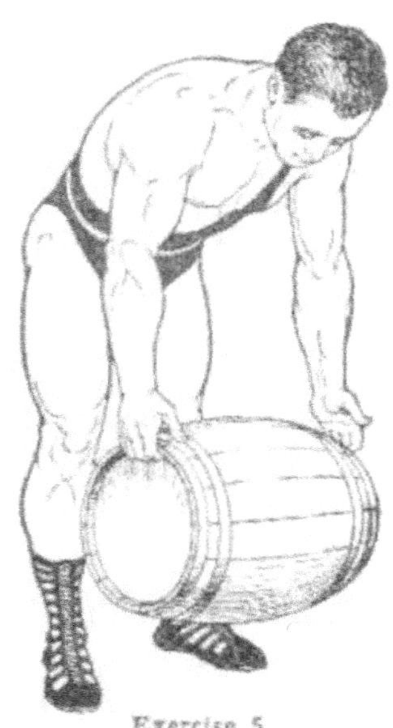

Exercise 5

Exercise 5

1. This is distinctly a grip lifting exercise. The man is gripping the chines (the name given to the edges of barrels).
2. The object of this exercise is to keep your legs and your back straight, and then lift it off the floor as high as you possibly can.
3. After that, place the barrel onto the floor and straighten out your fingers, then repeat this grip a few more times.

BARREL DIGIT CARRY

Barrel Digit Carry

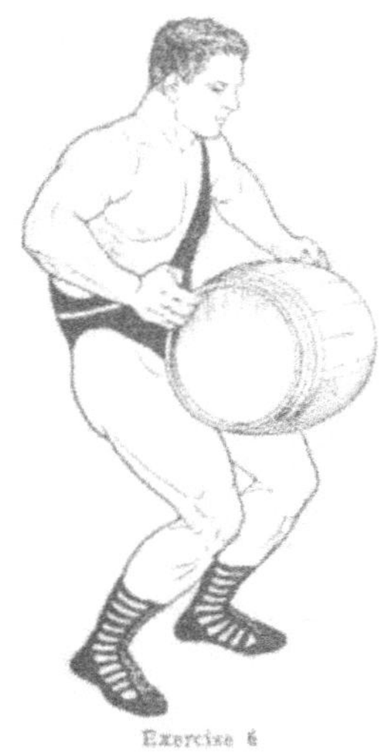

Exercise 6

Exercise 6

1. Lift the barrel up and onto the thighs.
2. Now practice this exercise (with exercise 5) several more times with a 100-lb. barrel. Remember to carry it by gripping the chines.

11

THE ROLLING FOREARM

The Rolling Forearm

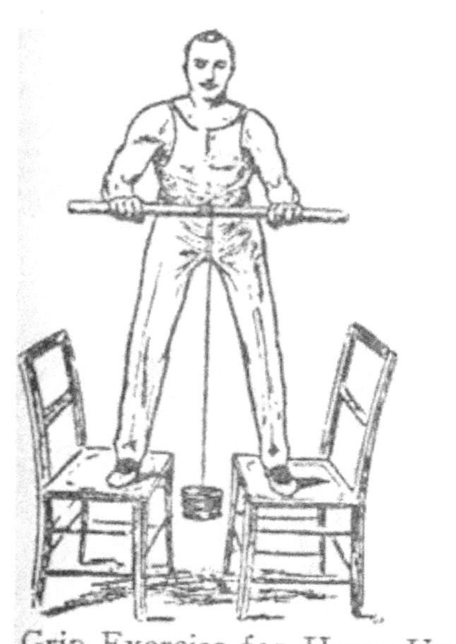

Grip Exercise for Home Use

Grip Exercise

1. Using a round stick, a thick broom-handle will suffice, but it should be from 1 inch to 1 and a 1/2-inches in thickness.

1. Make a hole through this and suspend a 5 lb. weight on a cord.
2. Standing on two chairs, holding the bar waist height, roll it with both hands, to coil up the cord. Do this both steadily and gradually.
3. Keep going until the weight is wound up closely, then unwind it to its full length. Do this winding and unwinding technique with continuous and reversal rolling, so as to get the most out of the exercise. Continue until you can't do anymore.

12

BICEP/TRICEP CURLS

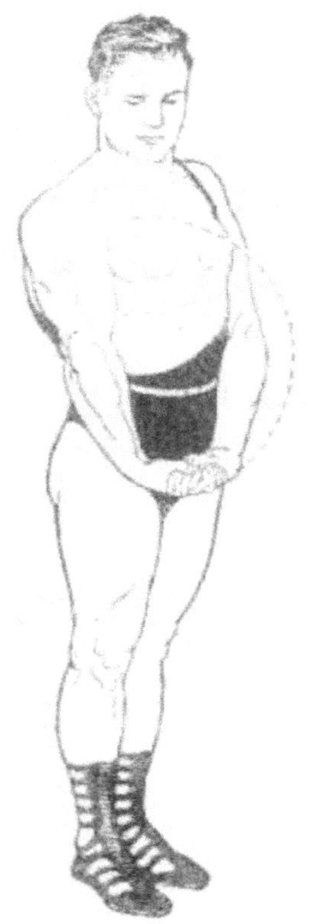

Bicep/Tricep Curls

Standing Exercise

1. Stand erect with your feet together.
2. Now, clasp the left hand in the right. Do this in front of your body with the palm of the right hand facing forward. Make sure the arms remain straight down, and by the sides.
3. Now, turn the right hand on the wrist upward, in a cupped motion so that the length between the hand and the place of the forearm is shorter.
4. Continue by bending the arm at the elbow, and then raise

your right hand (as if going) to the right shoulder. Throughout this part of the exercise, press down with the left arm hard, so as to resist the upward push of the right arm. When the right hand is curled to the shoulder, now allow the arm to return back to the starting position, but, resist the downward action, utilizing your strength by pulling up with the left hand.

5. Do this exercise and reverse the hands to develop both arms in equal proportions to one another. 6 reps to start, will suffice. You can do more later, as you require.

IN CONCLUSION

It's almost comical how much information has been suppressed due to corporate greed. This is just another one... in a list of so many. I mean who would have thought a man or woman would be able to bend steel? It still awes me when I watch Dennis Rogers bend a hammer in half or a video of Alexander Zass carrying a horse over his shoulders. With every new year, there comes new evidence which is shone on how truly amazing the human body is.

As with all things worthwhile in life, they all take time. With great patience and determination, you will also have the strength of these legendary men who I've had the pleasure of speaking about, above. As I said before, the workouts are easy, and they do not require much equipment, nor do they take strenuous hours to complete. And you can be the superman you always wanted to be...

I wish you so much success in your future endeavors, God bless, *Vince.*

P.S. If you want to learn some more amazing isometric exercises, just sign up to my newsletter, because there, I'm sharing another 27 isometric exercises including: the 8 isometrics exercises Bruce Lee used to practice on a daily basis! As well as loads of resources for you. So, if you think being stronger will help you in any area of your life, whether it be sports or any other aspect, then Click here sign up today. You won't be disappointed! I'll see you soon!

OLD TIME STRONGMAN

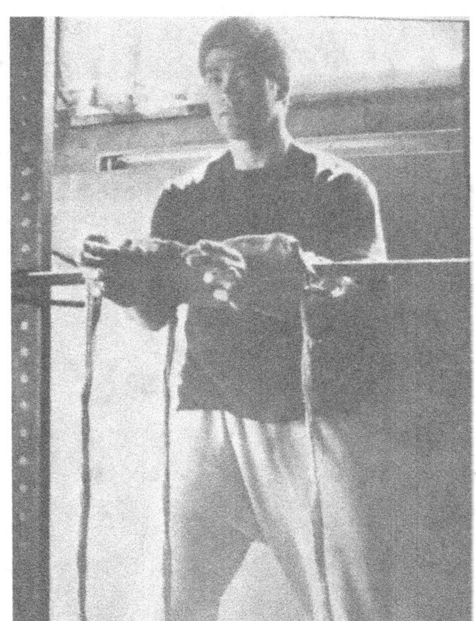

Bruce Lee pushing against a unmovable bar

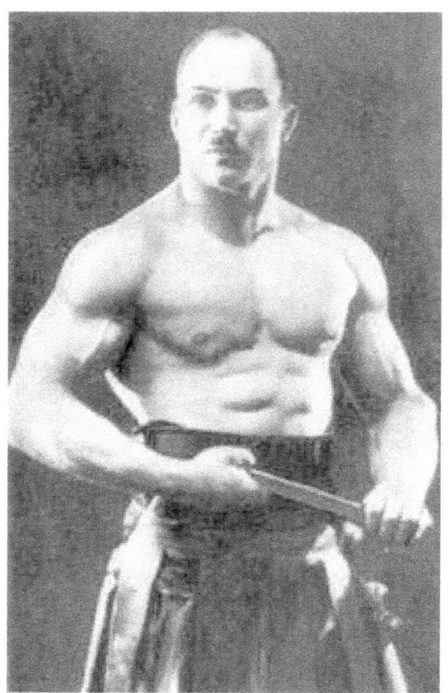

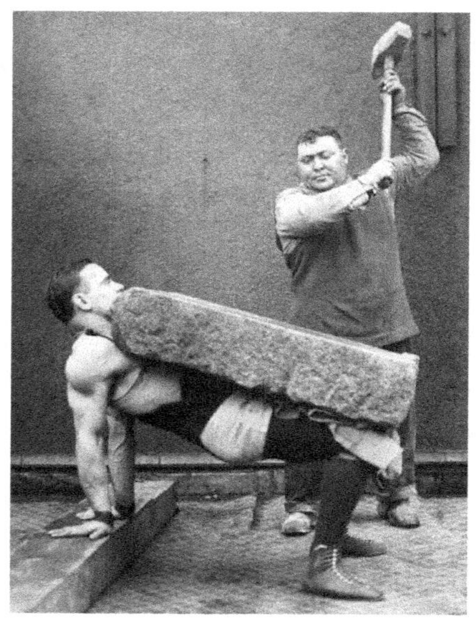

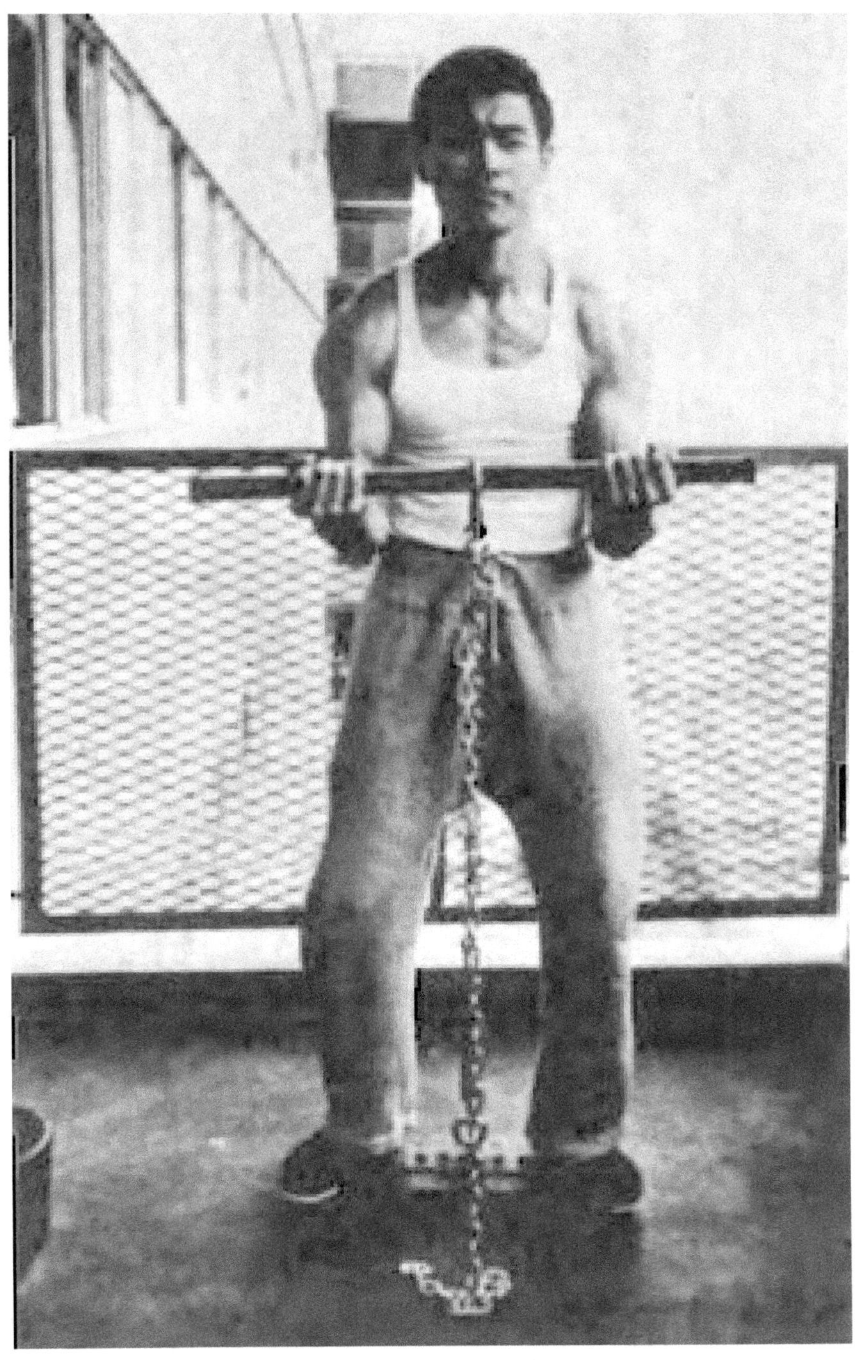

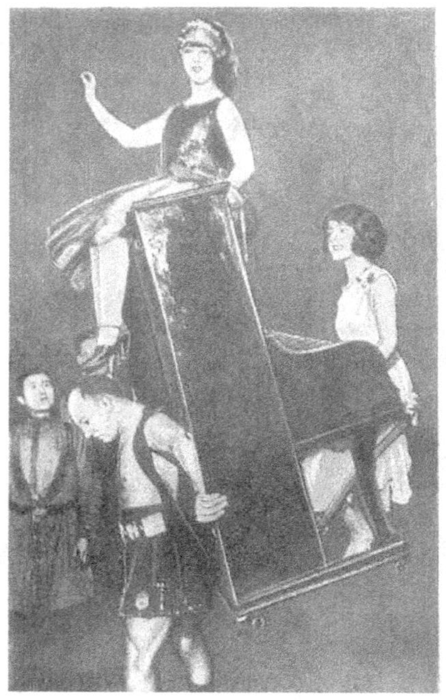

Alexander Zass

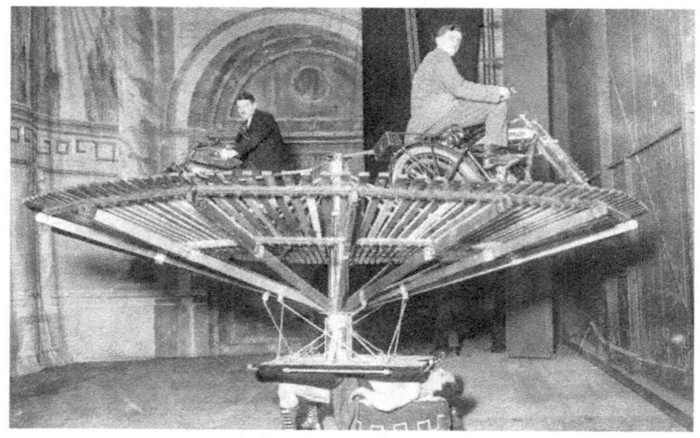

Siegmund Breitbart - motordrome on his chest

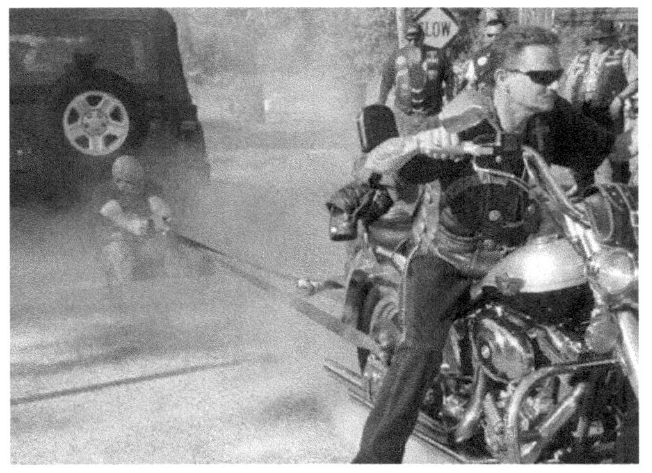

Dennis Rogers holding back a motorbike

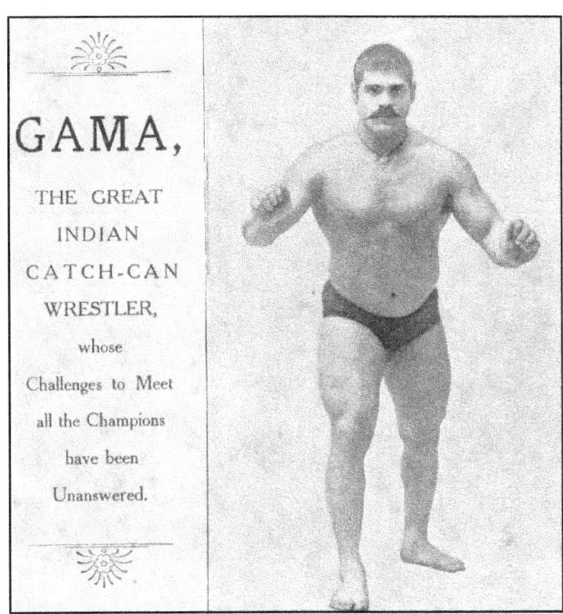

Vintage Great Gama promotion

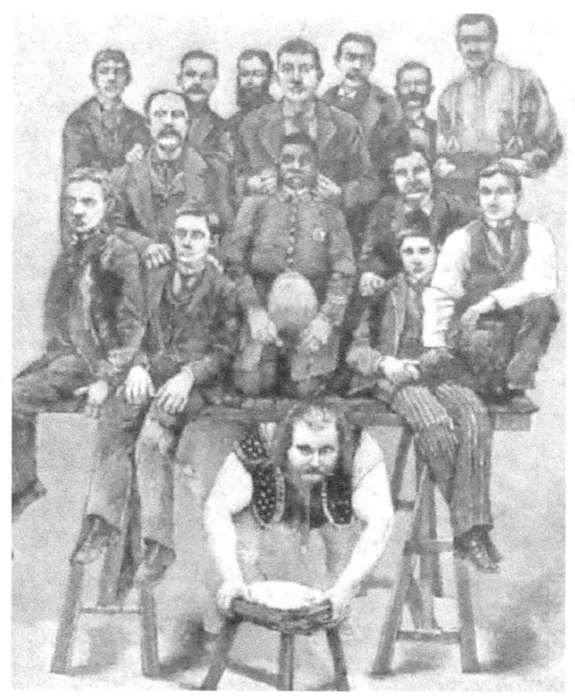

Louis Cyr

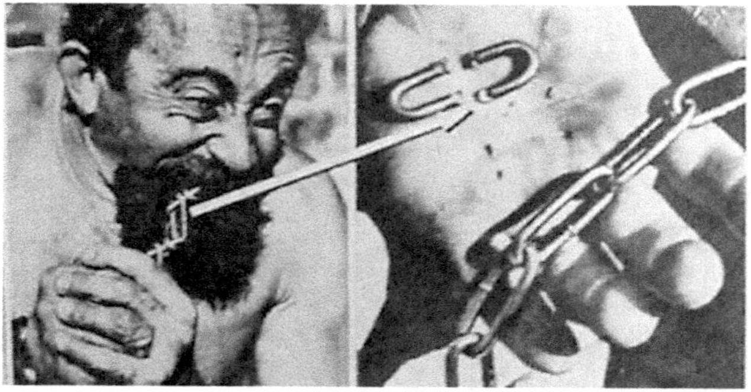

The Mighty Atom Biting a steal chain in half